T0171575

Travel Smart, Live Wise

Travel Smart, Live Wise

AN INSIDER'S GUIDE TO HEALTHY TRAVEL AND LIFESTYLE

STEPHANIE A. COLEMAN

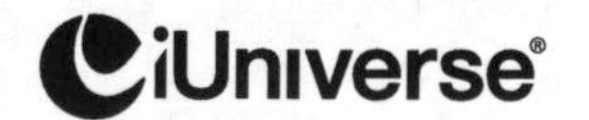

Travel Smart, Live Wise
An Insider's Guide to Healthy Travel and Lifestyle

Copyright © 2012 by Stephanie A. Coleman

All rights reserved. No part of this book may be used or reproduced by any means, graphic, electronic, or mechanical, including photocopying, recording, taping or by any information storage retrieval system without the written permission of the author except in the case of brief quotations embodied in critical articles and reviews.

iUniverse books may be ordered through booksellers or by contacting:

iUniverse
1663 Liberty Drive
Bloomington, IN 47403
www.iuniverse.com
1-800-Authors (1-800-288-4677)

Because of the dynamic nature of the Internet, any web addresses or links contained in this book may have changed since publication and may no longer be valid. The views expressed in this work are solely those of the author and do not necessarily reflect the views of the publisher, and the publisher hereby disclaims any responsibility for them.

Any people depicted in stock imagery provided by Thinkstock are models, and such images are being used for illustrative purposes only.

Certain stock imagery © Thinkstock.

ISBN: 978-1-4620-1302-9 (sc)
ISBN: 978-1-4620-1300-5 (e)

Print information available on the last page.

iUniverse rev. date: 07/08/2016

CONTENTS

Preface

My name is Stephanie Coleman. I was born and raised in Chicago, Illinois. I have been a flight attendant for United Airlines since 1970. It has been a wonderful and fulfilling career. As with all good things, there have been some downsides. In the early days, when I was junior, I missed important family gatherings, fun times with earthbound friends and events at my church, as well as a wedding or two. I am sure that, as a single parent, I have been absent for a few of my son's important dates. All in all, I have enjoyed seeing so many fascinating places, that most of my peer group have not experienced. Upon earning seniority, the flexibility of schedules and the increased variety of destinations have been wonderful.

I have learned a great many things through my travels. Experiencing different cultures and peoples and their customs, has been quite enlightening. As a black female from the south side of Chicago, I have been exposed to different foods, languages, and political thoughts. I feel truly blessed to have chosen this vocation.

I have always had an interest in athletics and health issues. I always thought of myself as healthy and fit, so when I was diagnosed with breast cancer in 2001, I was shocked. After learning more than I ever wanted to know about the disease and how cancer patients were treated, I vowed to learn as much as I could about preventing any further episodes of that disease and any others that might be a threat to me or others.

I have become a certified health consultant, a certified reflexologist, and a certified natural health professional. I want to learn as many modalities as I can before my life is over. I want to share whatever I learn with as many folks as I can. My purpose in writing this book is to do just that.

Acknowledgments

I would like to thank the good Lord for leading me to listen to a radio program called *Healthline.* This program stars Dr. Robert Marshall, CEO of Premier Research Labs, who answers folks' health questions. Through him I met a woman he had trained for eight years as a quantum reflex analysis practitioner. Her name is Mia Scheid. She has been my mentor, teacher, and friend since 2006. I had been a cancer survivor since 2001 at the time of our meeting. I felt pretty good, but knew I could feel better. I had been praying for guidance about my future vocation and use of my talents. Through Mia, I found some answers. With her encouragement and support, I believe I have found my way.

Mia Scheid of Fitness Arts has been a very positive influence in my life. Her wisdom and knowledge of life and health have made an indelible impression on me. Knowing her has enhanced my life and has given me a sense of purpose and hope for my future that I've never experienced before.

My son, Gregory Coleman, has always been in my corner, encouraging me in whatever direction I headed. I have never known anyone more focused. I hope his determination and discipline will rub off on me.

I would also like to thank my nephew, Justin Poindexter, and my friend Marilyn Broady, for helping me to overcome my computer phobia. They have helped me to come into the twenty-first century in regard to electronics.

My Brazilian friend, Izabel Harris, has given me words of encouragement and has shared her editing skills and computer skills with me.

I really owe a debt of gratitude to all the flight attendants and pilots I have come in contact with over the years. Our mutual love of flying, the camaraderie we feel, and the common suffering we share have been the main reasons for my writing the book. I pray this book will help them as much as they have helped me.

INTRODUCTION

Regular air travel can take a toll on the human body. Those of us who frequently travel by air need to be armed with as much accurate, concise information as possible, in order to stay healthy and limit disease. I have accumulated a mountain of information, which has been condensed here so that I can help those of us who travel frequently. Much of the information in this book is also applicable to the general public. The knowledge will be useful to all people seeking good health throughout their lives, but I am writing this book in particular to aid people who are employed in the travel industry and other frequent travelers.

The only investment that will pay dividends in the future is the investment in our health. According to an article by the Kaiser Family Foundation, it is estimated that seventy-six million Americans will turn sixty years of age between 2011 and 2014, and 53 percent of those people are chronically ill.[1] According to statistics from www.healthcareproblems.org, the average American man and woman spend the last three years of their lives using up all their savings on health care and nursing homes.[2]

Moreover, according to the AOA (Administration on Aging) "Retirees will need an estimated $635,000 per couple over age sixty-five to cover health care costs in retirement." [3] The Kaiser Family Foundation states that "Approximately 50 percent of personal bankruptcies in 2008 resulted from medical expenses."[4] And the statements at healthcareproblems. org says that 45 percent of adults report having problems paying medical bills.[5]

The number of uninsured people has grown 60 percent to twenty-five million from 2008 to 2011.[6] The fastest-growing segment of the underinsured population is from middle- and upper-income families.[7] The number of underinsured people among those with incomes of $40,000 or more tripled from 2008 to 2011, to 11 percent.[8] The World Health Organization says that, as of 2008, the highest rate of underinsured people (31 percent) in the United States is in families with incomes under the poverty level of about $20,000.[9] The amount people pay for health insurance increased 30 percent from 2001 to 2005, while incomes for the same period of time only increased by 3 percent.[10]

Life expectancy at birth in the United States was an average of 78.14 years in 2011.[11] The United States ranked forty-seventh in highest total life expectancy, compared with other countries.[12] The United States ranked forty-third among nations in infant mortality in 2011, down from twelfth in 1960 and twenty-first in 1990.[13] In 2007, 75 percent of total health care spending in the United States went toward treatment of chronic disease such as diabetes and asthma.[14] Approximately half of all chronic diseases are linked to preventable problems, including smoking, obesity, and physical inactivity.[15]

The Employee Benefit Research Institute reported in 2010 that 25 percent of employed people chose jobs based on health care provided.[16] Many cohabiting couples are now getting married in order to provide health care for the uninsured partner.[17] If these statistics are not enough to make people take better care of their health, I don't know what *is*.

I have been a flight attendant for over thirty-seven years. I have seen the travel industry go through many changes, some good and some not so good. I have experienced the decline of my own health, as well as the disproportionate decline of the health of many of my colleagues.

As a group, flight attendants and frequent fliers are exposed to myriad chemical toxins and poor air conditions, including recycled air and chemicals shipped in baggage requiring the pilot's signoff, and also to radiation. It is estimated that we are exposed to one thousand times more radiation on a cross-country flight than a person on the ground is exposed to. It is easy to understand why there are many reports of cancers among airline workers. Flight attendants are exposed to dangerous things, such as toxic materials transported on our aircraft, poor air quality, toxic cleaning agents, and increased radiation exposure. It is estimated that a flight from New York to Los Angeles gives you as much radiation as a normal person standing on the ground receives in a year.

Now that we know the dangers, what precautions can we take? Did you know that there are supplements you can take to mitigate the effects of radiation and the effects of environmental toxins? In this book, you will discover many simple and inexpensive ways to stay healthy in a world that can cause radical breakdown of our physical health. For example, one of the chapters in this book discusses the benefits of the antioxidants in green tea, which are effective in eliminating radiation effects.

It was about 1994 that I began flying international routes. I had been flying from Chicago to the west coast pretty regularly and was extremely excited at the change in destinations. I did notice, however, that my friends who started flying international routes before me seemed to be aging at an accelerated pace. They seemed very lethargic, somewhat disoriented, and most of them had put on about twenty pounds. I wondered if that would to happen to me.

Long story short, I gained about twelve pounds, was tired a great deal of the time, and in 2001, I developed breast cancer. I have been cancer-free since 2002. I have tried to learn as much as I can about keeping my body healthy.

In preparation for this book, I asked my flying partners and passengers what their concerns were about flying. A lot of folks had concerns about not eating good foods and not getting proper rest. Some people said they had gained many unwanted pounds as a result of traveling regularly. Some folks complained of varicose veins, constipation, indigestion, carpal tunnel syndrome, hearing loss, and insomnia. I will address most of these issues in this book.

In all my learning about health issues, there seems to be agreement in the material I have found that there are six principles to health and longevity. The longest-lived peoples on the planet all seem to be successful by following these steps:

1. Live in a nontoxic environment.

2. Be alkalized; have a proper pH balance in your digestive system.

3. Be well hydrated.

4. Be sure to get the minerals to support health, and eat healthy foods.

5. Exercise; be active.

6. Develop a positive attitude and have optimism for the future.

This book is designed as a road map to healthy living for individuals who travel by air frequently. Most of the information also applies to people who don't travel frequently. I will do the best I can to show how you can live a better life.

CHAPTER 1: LIVING IN A NONTOXIC ENVIRONMENT

To maintain a healthy external environment, you first need to be aware of all potential harm. You should understand that your skin is your largest detoxification organ. What most folks don't realize is that what you place on your skin is absorbed into your system. A lot of what you are exposed to in your environment is not under your control: gas emissions, weather toxins, pesticides, airplane fuel, and electromagnetic fields. However, there are some toxins you *can* control—things in your food and in your cosmetics, for example.

General guideline: If you cannot pronounce the ingredients in the lotions you use or in the food you eat, don't use or eat them.

* Many deodorants have aluminum, so you should not use them. Aluminum *is a metal used extensively in aircraft components, prosthetic devices and as an ingredient in antiperspirants, antacids and antiseptics.* [1] *Aluminum has been linked to Alzheimer's disease, currently afflicting 1 in 2 persons over the age of 70. Contamination may occur through the use of aluminum pots and pans, aluminum soda cans, and antiperspirants and other household items. Aluminum* can clog your lymph system and prevent

proper elimination of poisons from your body. You can find deodorants that don't have aluminum at most health-food stores.

* Although pharmaceutical companies want you to believe that it is good for you, *fluoride* is a poison. [2] It is best to use toothpaste that is fluoride-free. Most health-food stores offer toothpaste that does not contain fluoride.

* There are a great many cosmetics that have toxic ingredients. *Formaldehyde*[3] is commonly used in nail polish. Formaldehyde is also used as a disinfectant, a fixative, and a preservative. The EPA believes it to be a possible carcinogen; however, the FDA does not think it poses enough risk to necessitate regulation in cosmetics.[4]

* When combined with water, *lanolin* can cause skin rashes.[5]

* *Mineral oil* on the skin hinders respiration by repelling oxygen.[6]

* *Bentonite* is a kind of clay; when used in cosmetics, it may clog pores and, as a result, suffocate the skin.[7]

* *Talc* is a soft green mineral used in personal hygiene products and in cosmetics. Talc can cause lung cancer when breathed in.[8] It is used in the making of condoms and is used for diaper rash and genital hygiene. Talc has been known to cause uterine cancers.[9]

* *Salt* (sodium chloride) in most products can be very drying and corrosive.[10]

* *Animal collagen* is found in a lot of cosmetics. This product is made from ground-up animal carcasses, not something I want on my skin.[11]

* *Glycerin* is used as a solvent and tends to dry the layers of the skin.[12]

* *Alcohol* can cause body tissues to become more vulnerable to cancer-causing agents.[13] It is also very drying to body tissues.

Learn to read labels. If you can't pronounce the ingredients, think twice before buying the product. You can buy very good and helpful products at health food stores or online.

Table 1.1 lists some common food and cosmetic additives to avoid, in addition to the ones listed above. To help you understand Table 1.1, here are a few useful words:

* Excipient: Excipients are binders, fillers, and "glues" that are typically nonnutritive substances added to nutritional products. These substances often prove to be toxic.

* Neurotoxin: A neurotoxin is a poisonous complex that acts on the nervous system to damage or kill cells.

* Teratogen: A teratogen is a substance that can cause malformation of the developing embryo.

* Immune-compromising: Immune-compromising means that the substance can damage your body's immune system.

Table 1.1 Some Common Food and Cosmetics Additives, Their Uses, and Possible Problems Associated with Their Use

Substance	Uses and Problems
Magnesium stearate	A cheap lubricating agent; also used as a cosmetic colorant and uncaking and bulking agent; research shows it to be immune-compromising[14]
Methyl paraben	A benzoate family member; used in cosmetics and food; a known cancer-causing agent[15]
Microcrystalline cellulose	A cheap filler, used as a food additive to stabilize and thicken food it is made from wood pulp and used in machines to make tablets quickly. Would you eat wood pulp?[16]
Silicon dioxide	A cheap flowing agent, common sand; used as an anti caking agent in food. Silicon dioxide in food, when added externally in the right amount, can produce the intended effects, otherwise it may lead to severe health problems[17]
MSG (monosodium glutamate)	MSG is used as a food additive, also as a skin and hair conditioning agent; a well-known neurotoxin. MSG is "suspected" of causing compulsive eating.[18]
Methacrylic copolymer	Methacrylic acid, a component of the methacrylic acid copolymer, used as an artificial nail-builder, has been reported to act as a teratogen in rat embryo cultures.[19]
Triethyl citrate	Used as a deodorant, an antioxidant, and a plasticizer; can be considered harmful for its role in creating plastic, which does not break down[20]
Titanium dioxide	Used as a pigment (white) in toothpaste, skim milk, and medicines: liver toxin[21]
Cornstarch	Typically from cheap genetically modified corn; used to thicken and stabilize foods; absorb moisture in cosmetics; as a binder in tablets; can cause allergic responses[22]
Talc	Used in cosmetics as an abrasive, skin protectant, anticaking and bulking agent. A common excipient rarely listed on product labels; a suspected cancer-causing agent[23]

Dr. Robert Marshall class notes on Quantum Reflex Analysis. (2007)

Radiation [24, 25]

When we talk about our external environment and toxicity, as frequent fliers, we cannot ignore radiation. Most people think you can only be hurt by radiation from X-rays, toll booths, or chemicals.

Did you know that cosmic radiation levels are up to three hundred times higher at altitude than on the ground?[26] The Earth's atmosphere thins out at altitude, meaning flyers are exposed to higher levels of cosmic radiation. A typical cross country flight, for instance will give you about half the radiation you'd get from a chest x-ray. Three New York to Los Angeles trips in one month, would be close to three x-rays. While radiation might prompt cellular changes, this kind of exposure may only be a concern for flight crews, frequent flyers and pregnant women. Robert Souhami, of University College and Middlesex Medical School in London, has stated that radiation risk is dosage-related, so the more you fly, the greater the risk.[28]

Whether workers in the aviation industry are affected, however, is yet to be proven, though a number of studies have been carried out to investigate the biological effects of ionizing radiation on frequent fliers.[29] As with exposure to other forms of radiation, results have shown that exposure to cosmic rays could lead to genetic mutations in human egg cells and sperm cells, which could lead to complications when the fetus develops.[30]

Air Pressure

At an altitude of thirty-five thousand feet, within the aircraft, cabin pressure in a person's body cavities increases slightly. This commonly occurs in the ears and sinuses, which may lead to slight earache. If you suffer tooth decay, small cavities in the teeth can cause severe pain in flight. Also, keep in mind that the cabins low air pressure and your own inactivity can be an ugly one two punch that slows blood circulation, opening the door for deep vein thrombosis when blood coagulates to clog your veins. Women on birth control or with a family history of blood clots, should walk around for about five minutes every hour or so.

Air Quality

1. Air quality within the aircraft cabins can be poor, as the air-conditioning frequently recycles the air inside the cabin and fresh air isn't brought in. If people cough and sneeze within the cabin, it can cause passengers to suffer with minor colds and coughs. The plane's filtered, ultra-low humidity air can dry out your airways, stripping your nostrils of their protective mucous layer. Without that barrier, germs may have an easier time infecting your body's cells. Your best defenses are keeping your fingers out of you eyes and nose, and washing your hands often. It is also a good idea to boost your immune system a day or two before you travel by getting enough rest and eliminating as much stress as possible. You can also take Echinacea tincture 30-45 drops three times a day a week before travel for immune enhancing effects. Large doses of vitamin C will also help. You can also take soothing teas and of course chicken soup.

Jet Lag[31]

When our normal body clock is disrupted by traveling through different time zones, we are likely to experience jet lag. Jet lag results in disturbed sleep patterns, weakness, and disorientation. It's worse when we are traveling west to east, because the body finds it harder to adapt to a shorter day than to a longer day, and we lose hours as we move east. Our body clock is primed to respond to a rhythm of daylight and darkness. It is thrown out of sync when it experiences daylight at what it considers the wrong time, and it can take several days to readjust.

Your body clock is located at the base of the hypothalamus, which contains melatonin receptors.[32] The body clock receives information about light from the eyes, and it is also thought to receive input from that part of the brain which carries information about physical activities and excitement.[33] Melatonin is made in the pineal gland from tryptophan, and its synthesis and release are stimulated by darkness and suppressed by light.[34]

The secretion of melatonin is responsible for setting our sleep-wake cycle. The body clock is adjusted to the solar day by cues in the environment, such as light. These cues are called *zeitgebers*, or time givers. The main zeitgebers are the light-dark cycle and the rhythmic secretion of melatonin.[35] Exercise is thought to exert a weaker effect on the body clock than other time givers.[36] Although it is not yet completely understood, the body clock is believed to be partly responsible for the daily rhythms in core temperature and plasma hormone concentrations as well.[37]

Eastward travel is associated with problems in falling asleep at the destination bedtime and with difficulty arising in the morning. Westward travel is associated with early evening sleepiness and predawn awaking.[38] People traveling within the same time zone have fewer problems than those who cross several time zones. A time zone is about one thousand miles across. Jet lag can last several days. The number of days of jet lag is about two-thirds the number of time zones crossed for eastward flights and about one-half the number of time zones crossed for westward flights.[39] The American Academy of

Sleep Medicine says that older people tend to have fewer symptoms than younger travelers. They also state that exposure to the local light-dark cycle usually accelerates adaptation after jet travel across two to ten time zones.[40]

Signs of Jet Lag

Some of the signs of jet lag are the following: poor sleep, including delayed sleep onset (after eastward flights); early awakening (after westward flights); and fractionated sleep (after flights in either direction).[41] Other effects of jet lag can be poor performance of both physical and mental tasks during the new daytime; increased fatigue, frequency of headaches, and irritability; and decreased ability to concentrate.[42] Gastrointestinal effects (indigestion, diarrhea, constipation, and the altered consistency of stools) and decreased interest in and enjoyment of meals can also result from jet lag.[43]

Precautions Prior to Travel to Minimize or Avoid Jet Lag

* Stay healthy by continuing to exercise and eat a nutritious diet (although it requires high motivation and strict compliance with the prescribed light-dark schedules, meaning travelers should get on the local time zones as soon as they land).

* Break up the journey with a stopover.

* During travel, avoid large meals, alcohol, and caffeine.

* Drink plenty of water and move around the airplane to promote mental and physical activity. It is a good idea to wear comfortable shoes and clothing.

* Be sure to sleep during flights and avoid situations requiring critical decision-making, such as important meetings, on the day of arrival.

* Adapt to the local schedule as soon as possible. However, if the travel period is two days or less, travelers should remain on the home time. Optimize exposure to the local time.

* A few days before you travel, start getting up and going to bed earlier if you will be traveling east, or later if traveling west.

* During the flight, try to eat according to your destination's local time.

* Keep hydrated. Being dehydrated can intensify the effect of jet lag, especially after sitting in a dry plane for hours. Keep your fluid levels topped off with a cup of juice or water for each hour of the trip. Try to stretch during the flight.

* If you wear foam earplugs and a sleeping mask, you can cut down on disturbances to sleep onboard the plane.

* By controlling your exposure to daylight, you can trick your brain into beating the jet lag more quickly. As soon as you arrive, spend time outdoors in the daylight. This will regulate your body clock. Stay up till 11:00 p.m. when you arrive. Don't take a nap.

* Use sleeping remedies with caution. Sleeping medication is not recommended, as it doesn't help to adjust naturally to a new sleeping pattern.

Chapter 2: Keeping a Healthy Internal Environment

Keep Your pH Balanced[1]

One of the things we can do to insure good health is to keep our external and internal world as toxin-free as possible. This chapter is to inform you how to keep your internal world toxin-free.

From all the data I have acquired, it seems that keeping a proper pH in your body cells, the internal balance of acid vs. alkaline, is key to optimal health. pH stands for the power of H, or the amount of H+ ions (hydrogen ions) in a liquid. The pH scale ranges from 0 to 14. It measures the acidity or basicity of a solution. Pure water has a pH of 7, and is neutral. The higher numbers above 7 are basic, or alkaline. The lower numbers, below 7 are acidic. Your pH says a lot about your internal health. It tells how acidic or alkaline your tissues and fluids are. Everything living must remain in a certain pH range to function as designed. The human body likes to dwell around pH 7.4. [2]

The foods we eat leave a residue, or ash, after they're metabolized that is either acidic or alkaline.[3] The main acid generators are proteins, whether animal or plant.[4]

Dr. Otto Warburg received a Nobel Prize in the 1930s for his work on cell respiration. He found that disease cannot survive in an oxygen-rich environment.[5] Basically, diseased bodies were acidic at the cellular level, and disease is repelled by an oxygen environment. Having the proper pH balance in the body will repel disease.

When you have too much acid in your system, the brain mobilizes mineral buffers to raise the acidic pH of the internal environment in an effort to counteract the acids.[6] Buffers are the body's attempts, using alkalizing minerals and water, to combine with the acid to raise its pH before taking the acid out of the body by way of the kidneys.[7] The body loses these minerals along with the acid. These mineral buffers are often not sufficient to prevent damage to the kidneys.[8] As a backup, the kidneys start producing ammonia, which will raise the pH.[9] This can make your urine smell very strong and may create a burning sensation when you urinate. It's at this point that you may want to take cranberry juice for the pain. The ammonia smell indicates that you are deficient in minerals.[10] If you continue with this pattern of mineral deficiency, you can damage your kidneys.

Most people in the United States are mineral-deficient.[11] We are not getting the minerals from the foods we eat, because of the way this food is grown and the amount of chemicals, pesticides, etc., in the food. Our bodies don't make minerals. You can have the proper vitamins in your system to control the body's use of minerals, but if you don't have minerals, the vitamins have no function to perform. If you don't have minerals, the vitamins are useless.

You need adequate amounts of calcium, magnesium, and D3, a vitamin that aids in the absorption of calcium, to maintain the proper pH.[12] Here are some guidelines for calcium and D3 dosage, provided by womentowomen.com and hubpages.com/hub/vitamind3, respectively:

Calcium:

500 mg a day for children 1 to 19 years of age

1000 mg a day minimum if you are age 19 to 50

1200 mg a day if you are over 50 years of age

1500 mg a day for older adults

Vitamin D3:

400 IU per day for children

2000 iu for adults under 50 years of age

2000 iu per day for adults 50 to 70

2000 iu per day for adults over 70 years of age

I personally do better at 4000 iu per day

Magnesium: 150 mg a day

It is also recommended that you get at least twenty minutes of sunlight per day.[13] This habit feels good and is good for you, because the ultraviolet component of sunlight makes D3 in your skin.

Avoid Soft Drinks[14]

Think twice before you order that supersized drink. Our country has a love affair with soft drinks, but people need to be aware of the negative sides of soft drinks.

Soft drinks release sugar into the body, producing acids that tell the body food is on the way. If food is not forthcoming, this sets up an environment that is not helpful to the digestive system.[15]

Soft drinks have no nutritional value. Diet soft drinks are even worse, because they contain aspartame, which is known to cause cancer.[16] Heavy consumption of soft drinks can lead to obesity, kidney stones, heart disease, and diabetes.[17] Soft drinks also irritate the stomach lining and cause acid reflux. Soft drinks are called "diabetes in a can." The sugar dissolved in the liquid is quickly carried into the bloodstream, where its presence in overload quantities signals the pancreas to go into overdrive. The pancreas is a gland that produces enzymes to regulate blood sugar and fluids that help with digestion.[18]

The pancreas has no way of knowing if the sugar inrush is a single dose or the front end of a sustained dose. The assumption in the body's chemical controls is the worst-case scenario. To prevent nerve damage from oxidation, the pancreas pumps out as much insulin as it can.[19] Even so, it may not prevent nerve damage. But the heroic effort by the pancreas has a hefty downside. The jolt of insulin causes the body to reduce testosterone in the bloodstream and to depress further production of testosterone in both men and women.[20] Testosterone is the hormone that controls the depositing of calcium in the bones.[21] You can raise testosterone through weight-bearing exercise, but if you are chemically depressing it via massive sugar intake, then the body won't add calcium to the bones. Too much carbonation can also lead to calcium loss.[22]

Researchers have found that adults who drank one or more cans of soda a day, diet or regular, had a 50 percent higher risk of metabolic syndrome than people who didn't drink soda. Metabolic syndrome[23] is a cluster of risk factors, such as excessive fat around the waist, low levels of good cholesterol, high blood pressure, and heart disease, that indicate a risk for stroke, coronary artery disease, and type 2 diabetes.[24] If you must have a soft drink, know that it takes thirty-two ounces of water to dilute and overcome the effects of that soft drink.[25]

The caffeine in soft drinks is very bad for women who suffer from PMS (premenstrual syndrome). Caffeine may contribute to the bloating, headaches, and belly cramps that some women experience prior to menstruation.

According to celestialhealing.net/caffeine, emotional fatigue is another side effect of caffeine.[26] Caffeine wakes up the body, but it doesn't tell the body when to relax. Some folks suffer from panic attacks caused by caffeine; their hands become shaky, they perspire, and they can become paranoid.[27] According to en.wikipedia.org/wiki/caffeine, caffeine is a diuretic that can lead to dehydration, as it steals water from the body.[28]

Pregnant women should avoid foods containing caffeine, or should consume them only sparingly.[29] Caffeine increases risks of delayed conception, fetal growth retardation, and miscarriage.[30] Caffeine consumption can affect calcium balance and may contribute to decreased bone density and osteoporosis.[31] Caffeine can have behavioral effects, including anxiety, sleeplessness, addiction, and withdrawal upon cessation of consumption, in children as well as in adults.[32]

Quit Smoking[33]

All studies have shown that smoking is bad for the human body. The manufacturers of cigarettes state this bit of information on the product themselves. Smoking is the main cause of the cancers of the lung, voice box (larynx), mouth or oral cavity, throat (pharynx), bladder, and esophagus (the tube that connects the pharynx to the stomach).[34]

Smoking has also been linked to cancer of the pancreas, cervix, kidney, and stomach, and to some leukemias.[35]

Smoking can make asthma worse,[36] can reduce fertility, and can make for riskier pregnancies.[37] Smoking has been linked to birth defects and sudden infant death syndrome (SIDS).[38] Smoking can also cause blood clots or worsen blood flow in the arms and legs.[39] The longer men smoke, the more they risk erectile dysfunction.[40]

According the information collected to date, smokers shorten their life span by up to fourteen years.[41] Secondhand smoke is very harmful to those exposed to it.[42]

If you are a smoker, here are some changes to be aware of. Any of these could be signs of lung cancer or other conditions. If you experience these, get a medical checkup: new cough, any change in an existing cough, trouble breathing, weight loss, loss of appetite, hoarseness, wheezing, headaches, frequent lung or upper respiratory infections.[43]

There are more than four thousand different chemicals found in tobacco and in tobacco smoke.[44] Among these, sixty chemicals are known to be cancer-causing.[45] They include tar, cadmium, ammonia, and carbon monoxide, to name a few. If you have not quit this horrible habit yet, please be sure you take the recommended daily allowance (RDA) doses of vitamin C (3000 mg); selenium (50–200 mcg); and vitamin E (30 IU).[46]

Menthol cigarette smokers tend to hold the smoke in their lungs longer than smokers of unscented cigarettes.[47] "Light" cigarette smokers tend to inhale more deeply than smokers of regular cigarettes.[48] The so-called "light" cigarettes also have more chemical additives than regular cigarettes.[49] I know smoking a hard habit to break, but please try everything you can to quit. Quitting will surely improve your quality of life.

Get Enough Sleep

Travelers' sleep habits are disrupted by time changes when they cross time zones. It is important to get adequate sleep while traveling. We all know that performance is affected by lack of sleep. Ideally, it would be great to get seven to eight hours of sleep each night.

Our bodies operate in natural cycles. It is advisable not to disrupt these cycles. Everyone needs a minimum of five hours of uninterrupted sleep. With five hours, your body can produce adrenalin for the following day.[50] Each time you don't get five hours of sleep, your body may suffer from a lack of adrenalin. We need this hormone for quality of life. Adrenaline is the hormone produced by the adrenal glands, located on the top of each kidney. Also known as epinephrine, adrenaline is what is known as a catecholamine and is a key component in the stimulation involved in the "flight or fight" response. Adrenaline can act on many cells in the body, and it also can be used as a neurotransmitter when it is synthesized by specific classes of nerve cells in the nervous system. It is the actions outside the nerves that generate the characteristic response of the body to adrenaline.

Adrenaline acts on muscle and liver cells to break down the complex storage carbohydrate glycogen and release extra glucose into the blood-stream—a much more readily available source of energy. Acting on the cells in the digestive tract, adrenaline causes a reduction in digestive secretions and acts on the blood vessels to shunt blood away from the gut and toward the brain, heart, lungs, and muscles. Adrenaline also has a direct effect on the heart and lungs, stimulating the heart rate and the overall force of contraction of the heart muscles, widening the airways in the lungs so that oxygen absorption can be enhanced.

The brain is activated by the daily rising and setting of the sun, which triggers the release of chemicals and hormones that make us sleepy as darkness falls, and wakes us up with the sunrise. Scientists call this daily cycle our *circadian rhythm*. Things that disrupt this rhythm include worry, stress, illness, age, and traveling across time zones. These things can all result in insomnia, the inability to fall asleep or to stay asleep.[51]

You can help yourself sleep better if you can get into a routine of going to bed at the same time each night. Try to eat your last meal three to four hours before retiring. Eat more fresh fruits and vegetables and cultured foods, like kefir, yogurt, and sour kraut. Walk or exercise daily, and get plenty of sunshine. Eating too close to retiring for bed can strain your digestion and affect sound sleep.[52] Avoid caffeine, soft drinks, and alcohol after 2:00 p.m. Avoid food that is difficult to digest, like red meat. Also try to avoid MSG, aspartame, and preservatives, which stress the liver and can cause sleep problems.[53]

For pituitary and pineal gland support, you might want to take melatonin before sleep. In oriental medicine, the liver and gallbladder are key meridians that influence the head area.[54] Traditional Chinese medicine recognizes a subtle energy system by which chi is circulated through the body. This transportation system is referred to as a system of channels, or meridians. According to worldofchinesemedicine.com, there are twelve main meridians in the body—six yin and six yang—and each relates to the organs. To better visualize this concept of chi and meridians, think of a meridian as a riverbed over which water flows and irrigates the land—feeding, nourishing, and sustaining the substance through which it flows. (In Western medicine the concept would be likened to the blood flowing through the circulatory system.) If a dam were placed at any point along the river, the nourishing effect that the water had on the whole river, would stop at the point the dam was placed. The same is true in relation to chi and the meridians. When chi is blocked, the rest of the body that was being nourished by the continuous flow now suffers. Illness and disease can result if the flow is not restored. Toxicity in either energetic pathway can result in sleep problems. Heavy metals from dental work can create an acidic pH and a poor ability to rest.[55]

Your sleep area needs special attention. Your bedding should not be too hard or too soft. Synthetic bedding is not good for the body. Your sleep area should be quiet and dark. Too much light in the room, or leaving the radio or TV on, is detrimental to good sleep. These days we also have to beware of electromagnetic fields. An electromagnetic field is a physical field produced by electrically charged objects. It affects the behavior of charged objects in the vicinity. According to www.Mercola.com an electromagnetic field comes from power lines, home wiring, airport and military radar, substations, transformers, computers and appliances and can cause brain tumors, leukemia, birth defects, miscarriages, chronic fatigue, headaches, cataracts, heart problems, stress, nausea, chest pain, forgetfulness, cancer and other health problems. Be careful to read labels on your medications, to be sure that they do not interfere with sleep.

There have been a number of studies by the military to find out the minimum amount of sleep needed to produce enough adrenalin for proper function. They came up with the answer of five hours' worth of uninterrupted sleep per night.[56] If you awaken and realize you have only slept four hours and forty minutes, you should not raise your head more than 45 degrees above the rest of your body for twenty minutes more, or your body won't make the proper amount of adrenalin, as raising your head higher will reset the production of adrenalin back to zero.[57] It is preferable to get seven to nine hours of sleep, but if you can't get that many, try for five hours.

Take Green Tea

One way to get rid of your internal toxins is to ingest green tea to pull radiation out of your system, or detoxify your body.

The best information I have obtained about green tea is from Nadine Taylor, MS, RD, who wrote a book on green tea.[58] I will quote her, because she has the best explanations I have found on antioxidants. I want this book to be laymen-friendly, for obvious reasons. Her information is found on GreenteaLibrary.com. According to Nadine Taylor, "unfermented tea leaves contain large amounts of *catechins*, which are powerful disease fighters and potent antioxidants. And green tea is the *only* natural source of large amounts of catechins."[59]

Antioxidants, found primarily in fruits, vegetables, and grains, are powerful natural weapons against heart disease, cancer, stroke, Parkinson's disease, Alzheimer's disease, and the effects of aging, among other things.[60]

You might be wondering why anything that's anti oxygen would be good for you! But antioxidants don't work against oxygen; they work against oxidation—the chemical reaction that turns bananas black, makes oil rancid, and is believed to be a major cause of disease.[61] The harm caused by oxidation is called oxidative damage; the substances that fight oxidation are called antioxidants.

Free radicals are loose cannons in the body. A free radical is an atom or group of atoms with at least one unpaired electron; in the body it is usually an oxygen molecule that has lost an electron and will stabilize itself by stealing an electron from a nearby molecule.[62] Oxidative damage is caused by free radicals, which are highly reactive, unstable molecules. Free radicals can be generated by exposure to UV rays, toxins, cigarette smoke, microbes, and other sources. But the most common source of free radicals is the oxygen molecule itself. It happens like this:

Oxygen typically roams around the body in pairs, in the bloodstream, and these double molecules share electrons,[63] but sometimes the pair splits and becomes two separate oxygen molecules, called singlet oxygen. Because singlet oxygen has been separated from its twin molecule, it ends up missing an electron. To compensate, it races off throughout the body in search of another electron that will make it stable again.

Singlet oxygen is a very active molecule. It doesn't just wait around for a spare electron to float by; it goes out and snatches one from another molecule. This upsets and destabilizes the "new" molecule, which, in turn, careens off in search of a replacement electron from a third molecule. The process of electron stealing repeats itself over and over, a chain reaction rocketing from one molecule to the next. Eventually, the stealing of electrons damages not only molecules, but cells, tissues, organs, and even entire body systems. The damage caused by free radicals like singlet oxygen is believed to be a major cause of cancer, heart disease, aging, and many other diseases or conditions.

Antioxidants to the rescue! Antioxidants like green tea's catechins work against electron stealing and oxidative damage by neutralizing and stabilizing free radicals. They do this by donating an electron, so that singlet oxygen and other free radicals no longer have the need to steal.[64]

Green tea has been proven to be great at pulling radiation out of the body.[65] Green tea is the most frequently drunk beverage on the planet. It has extraordinary anti-aging properties. In Japan, women drink more than the average amounts of green tea, and they are known for their low mortality rate and longevity compared with women of other countries.[66] Deaths from cancer are very rare in this group. Many survivors of the bombing of Hiroshima and Nagasaki after World War II drank at least six cups of green tea a day.[67] The polyphenols are compounds with antioxidant, antibacterial, and anticancer activity that are found in green tea and other foods and plants. Among the many kinds of polyphenols are catechins.[68] Catchins are astringent, water-soluble compounds that can be easily oxidized. Numerous studies continue to confirm that green tea polyphenols have powerful anticarcinogenic, cardioprotective, and antimicrobial actions.[69] Long story short, green tea can prevent cancers and prevent metastasis.

Sooner or later, almost all elderly people show signs of brain and cognitive impairment, even if they don't fall victim to Alzheimer's disease, Parkinson's disease, strokes, or other illnesses that affect the brain. Since green tea has been shown to protect against or diminish all of these conditions,[70] does that mean it can also protect the brain from cognitive dysfunction? There are animal studies that find green tea catchins can prevent oxidative damage to DNA in brain cells, reverse mental deterioration, improve memory-related learning, and reduce the buildup of the kind of plaque associated with Alzheimer's disease.[71]

It has been estimated that if you travel from New York to Los Angeles you are exposed to as much radiation as a person standing on the ground gets in a year's time.[72] Green tea can protect human cells against radiation damage.[73] Green tea can lower fat absorption, and it has a cholesterol-lowering effect. Japan has a much lower rate of Alzheimer's than other countries, probably due to green tea. There are a few brands of liquid green tea concentrate on the market that have no caffeine or fluoride; you should be able to verify this information by reading product labels' ingredient lists. The recipe for pulling out radiation is one-half teaspoon in a liter of water, for every 1,500 flight miles. Regular over-the-counter green tea has too much caffeine, and you would have to drink twenty cups to get the same effect you get with a half teaspoon of the liquid.

As a flight attendant, I flew to China three times a month. Each time I arrived after the fifteen-hour flight, I would feel so exhausted and sick that I would want someone to put me out of my misery. The first time I used the liquid green tea, I felt energized upon arrival. It was remarkable! If you have to travel by air, please try this.

Chapter 3: Being Well Hydrated

The Body's Need for Water

We all know that water is critical to life. It is involved in most chemical reactions in the body. Water helps the body regulate temperature. Our bodies need eight to ten eight-ounce glasses of water each day. Water suppresses the appetite and helps the body metabolize stored fat.[1] The kidneys need water to flush toxins from the body. Without water, your kidneys can't work at full capacity, thus some of their load is dumped onto the liver. If the liver has to do the kidney's job, it can't work on its own job. This means the liver will metabolize less fat; therefore, more fat is stored in the body, contributing to weight gain.[2]

Drinking enough water is the best way to prevent fluid retention. If your body does not get enough water, it thinks this is a threat to survival and starts to hold on to every drop,[3] and then water is stored in extracellular spaces. This shows up in the body as swollen feet, legs, and hands. Diuretics can help reduce swelling temporarily, but they only force out the stored water your body needs, along with essential nutrients.[4] Give your body the water it needs; only then will stored water be released. Drinking enough water helps restore normal bowel function.[5]

Testing in Japan has proven that drinking three or four glasses of water the first thing in the morning can be beneficial in treating disease. The method is to drink the water on arising, and then brush teeth, etc. Wait forty-five minutes before eating or drinking anything else. It is also recommended to drink warm water or tea with meals and after meals. If you drink cold water or other fluids after or with a meal, the cold fluid will solidify the oily stuff you have just ingested and[6]will slow down the digestion. Once this sludge reacts with stomach acid, it will break down and be absorbed by the intestine faster than the solid food and will line the intestine. Very soon this will turn into fat and can lead to cancer.[7]

It is a very good idea to drink warm water first thing in the morning. 8 Studies have shown that warm water first thing in the morning will flush the kidneys, help the bowels move regularly and naturally, and prepare the stomach for food by stimulating the glands on its' walls.

Symptoms of Dehydration

Not having enough water can cause labored breathing with exertion, and mental confusion, indistinct speech, difficulty concentrating, decreased blood volume, and decreased urinary output.[9] There can also be dry mouth, declining physical performance, muscle spasms, and wakefulness.[10]

Early symptoms of dehydration are as follows: fatigue, anxiety, headaches, constipation, intestinal cramps, depression, and irritability.[11]

Advanced dehydration symptoms are as follows: heartburn; rough, dry skin; nosebleeds; dry mucus membranes in eyes, nose and throat; joint and back pain; dark, strong-smelling urine; nausea, and colitis.[12]

Emergency symptoms of dehydration are the following: weak, irregular pulse; irrational behavior; shallow, rapid breathing; low blood pressure; type 2 diabetes; psoriasis; allergies; and asthma. [13] If you find yourself experiencing two or more of these symptoms, I would recommend you get to an emergency room quickly. You will probably need an IV to replace the electrolytes you have lost.

In order to test for dehydration, pinch the skin on the back of your hand. The speed at which the skin snaps back flat when you let go indicates the level of dehydration. If you are properly hydrated, the skin should snap back quickly. Dehydrated skin peaks and slowly returns to the flat of the hand.[14]

Chapter 4: Digestion and Healthy Foods

Why Digestion Is Important[1]

When we eat foods, they are not in a form that the body can absorb or use as nourishment. They must be broken down into tiny molecules that the body can use. Our food and drink must be changed into the smaller molecules of nutrients before they can be absorbed into the bloodstream and carried to the cells throughout the body. Digestion is the process by which food and drink are broken down into smaller parts. The digestive process starts with the brain. When we think of food, salivation and enzyme production begin in the mouth.

The Digestive System

The Mouth

The following section was presented in a core class on Nutrition by Elaine Newkirk ND, LPN,2008 she states;

"The mouth's job is to break food into smaller parts. The enzyme amylase breaks starches down into saccharides, or sugars. Chewing breaks food down into small pieces. At least 60 percent of carbohydrates are digested because of these enzymes in the mouth.[2]

The Stomach

A full stomach holds around 6.5 cups of mass.[3] The lining of the stomach is made up of three directional layers of muscle that expand and contract to mix food and digestive juices. Starch digestion that began in the mouth continues in the stomach if conditions are right.

Pepsin from the stomach, enzymes from the mouth, and enzymes from the food break the food down in the stomach. Within an hour after food enters the stomach, the protein and mineral bonds are broken by a process that uses hydrochloric acid. This prepares the nutrients to be absorbed in the small intestine. Some foods take longer to be absorbed. Fruits go through the system faster than other foods. On an empty stomach, fruits take about twenty minutes to be absorbed. Meats and other foods can take up to four hours to be digested. If hydrochloric acid is not present in the stomach due to a lack of raw materials, the protein and mineral bonds will not be broken and absorption will be hindered.

Most adults by about age forty produce only 25 percent of the hydrochloric acid they did when they were twenty.[4] By the time the average person reaches sixty years of age, he or she produces less than 10 percent of the hydrochloric acid that he or she produced at age twenty The hydrochloric acid not only is essential for digestion, but is also necessary to kill any bacteria, parasites, and viruses in the food that goes through the digestive system. It is highly recommended that you take digestive enzymes and hydrochloric acid supplements to successfully digest food.[5] I recommend all adults over the age of forty take digestive enzymes with their meals.

The Small Intestine

Your small intestines are fifteen to twenty-three feet long, depending upon your height.[6] The small intestines are lined with villi, the hair like protrusions that propel food through the intestines and absorb nutrients into the bloodstream.

There are three parts to the small intestine: the duodenum, the jejunum, and the ileum.

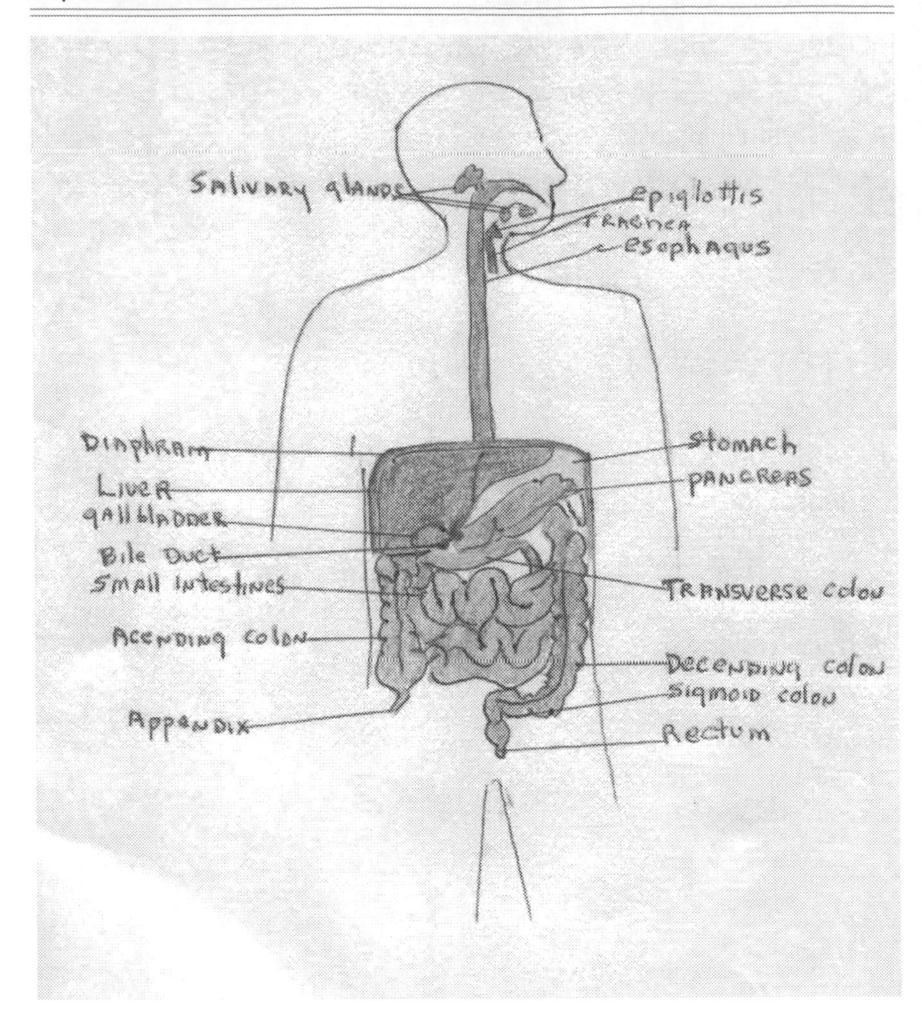

Figure 4.1 Diagram of the Digestive System. *Source:* http://www.annecollins.com/food-digestion-guide.htm

The Duodenum

The duodenum is the only part of the small intestine protected by a mucus lining. It is about ten inches long and is lined with glands that secrete an alkaline mucus that supports the intestinal enzymes and aids in the absorption of nutrients. Chyme, the partially digested semiliquid food that leaves the stomach, has a pH of about 1.5 to 3; it is very acidic, and must be rapidly alkalized by bile and pancreatic secretions.[7] Bile from the liver is stored in the gallbladder. The bile enters the duodenum to emulsify or break down fats and to alkalize the foods leaving the stomach. Some nutrients are absorbed in the duodenum.

Bile is made in the liver and is only stored in the gallbladder. The removal of the gallbladder does not stop the drip of bile. It simply slows the degreasing and alkalizing process.[8] The duodenum secretes hormones that stimulate the gallbladder, liver, and pancreas. The pancreas secretes enzymes that aid in digestion.

Minerals that look like baking soda enter the duodenum from the pancreas to complete the alkalizing process. It can take food four hours or more to go from the mouth past the duodenum, especially if the food is fatty.[9] The chyme moves on to the jejunum, the next part of the small intestine.

The Jejunum[10]

Pancreatic enzymes are made according to need. Complete digestion of chyme into minute particles is necessary before food can be used by the cells as nourishment. The pH in the small intestine must be at least 7.5 for pancreatic enzymes to do their job. The jejunum is the part of the small intestine where maximum absorption of digested food, minerals, and water into the blood takes place. It also acts as a path for digested food to pass to the large intestine for further water absorption.10

The Ileum

Most nutrient absorption occurs here, provided that proper chemical reactions have occurred in the previous steps. Proteins and peptides are broken down into amino acids in the ileum. Lipids are broken down into glycerol and fatty acids. Capillaries in the villi absorb amino acids, glucose, fructose, and galactose for the bloodstream, while lacteals, lymphatic vessels arising from the villi, transport fatty acids and glycerol to the lymphatic vessels.[11] A fungus often referred to as *Candida* or yeast lives here to digest any particles or carbohydrates that are too large to be nutritious, thus protecting the bloodstream from circulating food particles, which could cause allergies.[12] If food is predigested in the stomach, or digested in the intestines, the need for yeast is minimal. In the ileum, bile salts from the liver are absorbed. The end of the ileum connects -with the large intestine.

Large Intestine (Colon)

It is in the large intestine that remaining moisture is absorbed into the body as hydration through the walls of the bowel. The large intestines act as a processing and storage chamber for unused food and waste that awaits evacuation."

Elimination

"There are four routes of elimination from the body.

1. The bowel

2. The skin

3. The respiratory tract

4. The urinary tract

If one route is not working properly, the others have to work harder. Sister systems are the large intestines, the lungs, and the kidneys. Healthy bowel movements should occur two to three times daily and be soft, formed, and should happen without straining. Transit time from mouth to anus is twelve to eighteen hours. [13]

For the respiratory tract to work properly, correct deep breathing must occur. There must also be appropriate amounts of water for the urinary tract to work, about half an ounce per pound of body weight. The average human uses two liters of water just to breathe each day.[14]"

Dry brushing with a soft, natural bristle brush before showers cleanses and exfoliates the skin, allowing it to breathe.[15] This process should take five minutes and should be done at least three times weekly. Wearing natural fibers near the skin allows skin to eliminate properly. The body eliminates waste through perspiration. A strong odor to the sweat indicates nutrient deficiencies or food sensitivities. Some odors can be a result of medicines one might be taking.

Cycles of the Digestive System

The digestive system has three cycles:

Appropriation, noon till 8:00 p.m.

Assimilation and absorption, 8:00 p.m. to 4:00 a.m.

Elimination, 4:00 a.m. till noon

Appropriation time is when you should eat. Assimilation is when the food is used by the body and, you should not be eating then. Elimination is when waste materials are disposed of. It is best to eat only fruits during this time. Fruits go through your system {from mouth to bloodstream} within thirty minutes. All other foods can take anywhere from four to six hours. Taking in other foods during this time can significantly slow down the elimination process.[16]

Food Combining [17]

Flight attendants and other people who travel frequently find it difficult to eat well. As a result, healthy weight management is almost impossible. In order to establish a healthy body, we must learn the principles of food combining. Most people don't understand how the digestive system works. Our bodies have uncompromising requirements and limitations. Food combining is a system based on logic and on a realistic way of life. It honors and supports the body and its ability to achieve the best level of health possible when we allow it to do so.

It is a common yet wrong belief that the stomach is able to digest any number of different foods at the same time. Digestion is governed by physiological chemistry. It is not only what we eat that is important, but also how we assimilate it.

Digestive enzymes are secreted in specific amounts and at special times. Different foods require specific secretions. Proteins require the body to secrete different enzymes than the ones it secretes for breaking up carbohydrates or fats. When these different enzymes are mixed in the body, they tend to cancel each other out. Acid or gastric digestion cannot be carried on at the same time as an alkaline or salivary digestion. If you try to do them at the same time, before long, digestion cannot proceed at all. The rising acidity of the stomach soon completely stops carbohydrate digestion. According to Mia Scheid, CNC, from Fitness Arts, the best efficiency in digestion requires us to eat in such a way as to offer the least resistance to the work of digestion.

Table 4.1 Table of Food Combinations

Acid fruits = oranges, lemons, kiwi, grapefruit, strawberries, and any fruit with high acid content

Nonacid fruits = apples, pears, peaches, blueberries, and melons

Common foods	Combine well with	Combine badly with
Sweet fruits (sub acid or nonacid fruit) *See Chart 4. 1 for lists*	Sour milk	Acid fruits; starches (cereals, bread, potatoes); proteins except for nuts
Acid fruits	Other acid fruits	Sweets (all kinds); starches (cereals, bread, potatoes); proteins except for nuts
Green vegetables	All proteins	Milk
Starches	Green vegetables, fats, and oils	All proteins, all fruits, acids, and sugars
Meats (all kinds)	Green vegetables	Milk, starches, sweets, other proteins, acid fruits and vegetables, butter, cream and oils
Nuts (most varieties)	Green vegetables, acid fruits	Milk, starches, sweets, other proteins, butter, cream, oils

Eggs	Green vegetables	Milk, starches, sweets, butter, cream, oils, and lard
Cheese	Green vegetables	Starches, sweets, other proteins, acid foods, butter, cream, oils and lard.
Milk	Nothing; best taken alone	All foods
Fats and oils	All starches, green vegetables	All proteins
Melons (all kinds)	Nothing; best eaten alone	All foods
Cereals (grains)	Green vegetables	Acid fruits, all proteins, all sweets, milk
Legumes: beans and peas	Green vegetables	All proteins, all sweets, milk, fruit (all kinds) butter, cream oils, lard

Source of table: Mia Scheid, CNC, Mias@fitnessarts.net

Some Principles of Food Combining

1. Do not eat two concentrated proteins at the same meal. This means don't have eggs with meat or cheese with nuts. You should not have meat and milk, or eggs or nuts at the same meal.

2. Please don't eat fats and proteins at the same time. This means do not use fats like cream, butter, and oil with proteins like meat, eggs, cheese, and nuts. Fat depresses the action of the gastric glands in the stomach by delaying the development of appetite juices and preventing the pouring out of the proper gastric juices to digest meats,

nuts, eggs, or other proteins. During the ingestion of food, the stomach relaxes to accommodate the meal. Gastric tone exerts an emptying force delivering food from the stomach to the small intestine. Fats may lower the entire gastric tone more than 50 percent.

3. Do not eat a concentrated protein and a concentrated carbohydrate at the same meal. This means do not eat protein foods along with bread, cereals, potatoes, sweet fruits, cakes, etc. Candy and sugar greatly inhibit the secretion of gastric juices and markedly delay digestion. If these items are consumed in large quantities, they can depress stomach activity.

4. Carbohydrates and acidic foods should not be eaten at the same meal. Don't eat bread, rice, or potatoes (carbs) with lemons, limes, oranges, grape, pineapples, tomatoes, or other sour fruits. This is because the enzyme ptyalin acts only in an alkaline medium. It is destroyed by even a mild acid. Fruit acids not only prevent carbohydrate digestion, but also produce fermentation. Oxide acid, for example, diluted to one part in ten thousand, completely stops the action of ptyalin. There is enough acetic acid in one teaspoon of wine vinegar to halt salivary digestion. Tomatoes should also never be combined with starchy food, as the combination of the various acids in the tomatoes, which are intensified on cooking, is very much opposed to the alkaline digestion of starches. Tomatoes may be eaten with leafy vegetables and fatty foods. What all this means is that when folks say they cannot eat oranges or grapefruit as they give them gas, people could

be blaming the fruit, when the problem may be with the escape of starches and the body's release of pancreatic juice and intestinal enzymes to break them down. In cases where there is hyperacidity of the stomach, there is great difficulty digesting starches. Fermentation and poisoning of the body occurs, along with much discomfort.

5. Do not eat acid fruits with proteins. Oranges, lemons, tomatoes, pineapples, etc., should not be eaten with meats, eggs, cheese, or nuts. Acid fruits hamper protein digestion and result in putrefaction. Milk and orange juice, while by no means are an indigestible combination, is a far from good combination. Orange juice and eggs form an even worse combination.

6. Do not consume starch and sugars together. Jellies, jams, butter, honey, syrups, etc., on bread, cake, or at the same meal with cereals, potatoes, etc., will produce fermentation. The practice of eating starches that have been disguised by sweets is also a bad way to eat carbohydrates. If sugar is taken into the mouth, it quickly fills with saliva, but no ptyalin (which converts starch into sugar) is present, and ptyalin is essential for starch digestion.

7. Do not consume melons with any other foods. Watermelon, honeydew melon, cantaloupe, and other melons should always be eaten alone. This is possibly due to the ease and speed with which melons decompose.

8. Milk is best taken alone, if at all. Milk is the natural food of mammalian young; each species produces milk precisely adapted to the needs of its young. It is the rule that the young take milk alone, not in combination with other foods. Milk does is not digested in the stomach, but in the duodenum; hence, in the presence of milk, the stomach does not respond with secretions.

Fasting

Your body spends 80 percent of its energy each day in digesting food. Fasting at least one day a week is a very good practice. By fasting, you give your body a chance to work on repairing other parts or organs that may need some help. There are some effective, harmless fasts out there that anyone can utilize. Some folks like fasting with fresh juices for a day. I like to fast each Monday from the time I arise until about 6:00 p.m. I fill a liter of water with about six teaspoons of lemon juice, four teaspoons of organic maple syrup, and cayenne pepper to taste. This concoction is pleasant-tasting and good for detoxing the body. You could just drink plenty of water till 6:00 pm, but that's not as much fun or as tasty. You'll be surprised at how well you feel.

Chapter 5: Being Active.

The Importance of Exercise[1]

Regular aerobic exercise stimulates lymphatic drainage. Lymph vessels are the sewage system of the body. Lymph fluid is the intermediary between blood and bodily cells; in lymph, nutrients are exchanged and wastes are carried off. There is as much lymph fluid in the body as blood, but it must circulate without the benefit of a pump or heart. Exercise gives the lymph nodes and vessels the "massage" they need to keep them working efficiently. So the more you move, the better your system works.

Benefits of Exercise

* Weight management. People who exercise regularly are more likely to be at and to maintain a healthy body weight.

* Heart health. Exercise, especially aerobic exercise, strengthens the heart muscle, reduces the resting heart rate, and decreases the heart's workload. The changes that occur with exercise also help

lower blood pressure and increase HDL (high-density lipoprotein) levels in the blood.[2]

* Diabetes prevention and management. Folks with extra body fat are more apt to develop diabetes than people who don't have extra body fat. If you keep body fat within the normal range, aerobic exercise can decrease your risk of developing diabetes. Aerobic exercise will also help prevent overweight people from developing diabetes. Weight training and aerobic exercise increase the sensitivity of body tissue to insulin; this means the body needs to produce less insulin to keep blood sugar levels in check. Exercise can reduce or eliminate the need for medication to maintain blood glucose levels.

* Bone and joint health. Lifting weights helps maintain muscle size and strength. Weight-bearing exercise stimulates bones to become denser and stronger.

* Reduced cancer risk. There is evidence that people who exercise regularly reduce their risk of colon and breast cancers.

* Well-being. Exercise improves mood and overall feelings of well-being, because exercise increases the body's production of endorphins. Endorphins are thought to aid in relaxation, pain tolerance, and appetite control.

The Importance of Muscle

The average American woman loses eight pounds of muscle and gains twenty-three pounds of fat between ages twenty and forty years. The average man loses a quarter of total body mass between ages twenty and eighty years. (BMI, or body mass index, is an index of a person's weight in relation to his or her height, not his or her body composition.) His immunity seems to go right down the drain with it. Stored body fat is very inactive metabolically and burns very few calories. It sits like dead weight, waiting to be used up for fuel. Muscle is always in motion. Opposing muscles are in constant tension to hold up your skeleton and to enable you to make every movement you make. Muscle is the engine of your body, in which almost all your energy is created, by burning fats, carbs, and proteins.[3]

The bottom line is that we need the muscle we have and cannot afford to lose any more by cutting down too much on calories or exercising for extended periods of time above our target heart rate. According to mayoclinic.com, target heart rate, or training heart rate, is described as a desired range of heart rate reached during aerobic exercise—a rate at which the heart is exercised but not overworked. This theoretical range varies from person to person and is based on one's fitness level, age, and physical condition. The THR can be calculated by using a range of 50 to 80 percent intensity. Calculating the target heart rate requires knowing one's maximum heart rate. This number may be calculated by subtracting one's age in years from the number 220. So according to this equation, a thirty-nine-year-old would have a maximum heart rate of 181.

Low-intensity workouts burn a higher percentage of calories from fat, while high-intensity workouts burn a lower percentage of calories from fat.[4] Translation: exercise does not have to be vigorous to be effective.

Walking may be the best form of exercise to start out with. Walking burns fat, requires no special equipment, and proves less stressful than other forms of exercise. Thirty minutes a day is quite effective.

Swimming is low-impact, with as many benefits as walking, and may be more comfortable for folks with back or joint problems.[5] However, swimming doesn't have the weight-bearing effects that walking has, so it's not as good for people with osteoporosis or osteopenia.

Done correctly, weight training is the most efficient and safest form of exercise there is. Weight lifting need not be a power sport. It's good to start with one- or two-pound weights at first and then gradually increase the resistance. Remember, it's never too late to start building muscle. Working out with weights increases walking ability, prevents broken bones, gives pain relief, and results in improved sleep, decreased depression, and greater ease in performing activities of daily living. Working with weights increase muscle mass, decreases insulin levels, and promotes the release of human growth hormone (HGH).

It is important to know what HGH is and what it does in the body. HGH is produced in the pituitary gland. It promotes growth in children and plays an important role in adult metabolism. It repairs tissue, promotes growth, mobilizes fat stores and the use of fat, and shifts the metabolism to the preferential use of fat. (It is ideal to burn fat, and not muscle, for fuel or energy.) The amount of human growth hormone that the body produces declines with age. The production rate of HGH is reduced by half by age sixty. The type of exercise that has the most effect on the release of HGH is weight training.

The process works like this: as we lift weights, the straining muscles develop microscopic tears. This calls for HGH to repair them and stimulates growth of new muscle fibers to increase those with the damage. While the tissue building is in progress, the HGH converts the muscles into tiny fat-burning ovens. HGH also promotes the release of fat from fatty tissue to ensure that the new muscles receive a steady supply of fuel. Building muscle is the best, fastest way to sculpt the body.

Aerobic fitness is extremely beneficial and should be combined with weight training. It's best to perform aerobic activity before weight training. You should always stretch before exercise, to maximize your HGH release. Exercise on an empty stomach and stay away from simple carbs before your workout. Once you become more advanced, work each body part once a week. Muscle takes about forty-eight hours to break down worn cells, and then about forty-eight to seventy-two hours to build new, stronger replacements. That's a total of five days. From days five to eight, strength remains at maximum and then slowly declines. So exercising a muscle every five to eight days is an optimum program for success. Do three sets of twelve reps (repetitions) of each exercise. By the time you reach rep number ten, you should really start to feel the "burn." When your twelfth rep becomes too easy, it's time to increase the weight. Make sure you drink plenty of water to prevent dehydration. Make sure you're taking enough minerals, vitamins, and supplements to support your newly active body. (Note: please remember that it is always a good idea to get a complete physical checkup before beginning any exercise program.)

Exercise helps to:

1. Eliminate unwanted fat

2. Prevent cancer

3. Lower cholesterol

4. Reduce blood pressure

5. Strengthen heart and lungs

6. Reduce depression

7. Protect against diseases

Body Types

There are three basic body types (somatotypes): ectomorph, endomorph, and mesomorph. A person can be a combination of any of the three types. A great many folks are a solid one or the other. Each body type has unique characteristics. Each type has different exercise requirements. Below is a chart showing how each type looks, along with body characteristics.

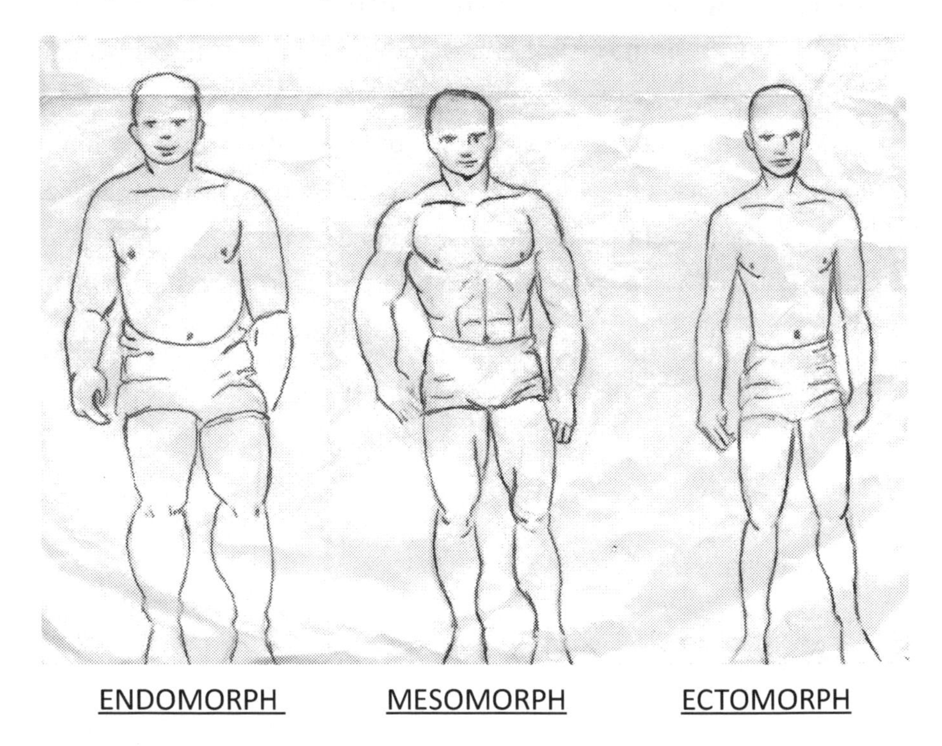

Figure 5.1 The Three Basic Types

Table 5.1 Body Type and Characteristics

Physical Characteristics

Ectomorph	**Endomorph**	**Mesomorph**
Thin, flat chest	Soft body	Hard, muscular body
Delicate build	Underdeveloped muscles	Overly mature appearance
Youthful appearance	Round shape	Rectangular shape
Lightly muscled	Overdeveloped digestive system	Thick skin
Large brain		Upright posture
Stoop shouldered		

Personality Traits

Self-conscious	Love of food	Adventurous
Introverted	Tolerant, sociable	Desire for power and dominance
Inhibited, artistic	Love of comfort	Assertive, bold
Mentally intense, nervous	Relaxed, enjoys affection	Zest for physical activity
Emotionally restrained	Good-humored	Love of risk and chance

Examples of ectomorphs are marathon runners, basketball players, and fashion models. Examples of endomorphs are sumo wrestlers, offensive linemen, and defensive linemen in the NFL. Examples of mesomorphs are running backs, boxers, and sprinters.

Ectomorphs should do thirty-to-forty-five-minute sessions of cardio at least four or five times per week. Ectomorphs should strength-train three or four times per week, lifting light to medium weights, and doing medium to high reps.

Endomorphs need twenty-to-thirty-minute sessions of cardio work, two or three times per week. Their strength training should consist of two to four short (thirty-minute) workouts per week.

Mesomorphs need more cardio, thirty-to-forty-five-minute sessions three or four times per week. Strength training for mesomorphs should be forty-five to sixty minutes, three or four times a week. They can use light, medium, and heavy weights for low medium and high reps. The type of weights depend upon the person's goals.

CHAPTER 6: HAVING A HEALTHY MENTAL ATTITUDE: YOU ARE WHAT YOU THINK

According to Phillip Day in *Health Wars*, studies done of the longest-lived cultures on the planet (i.e., those cultures that live longest) have discovered that they have some things in common.[1] The cultures that have the healthiest people also have some things in common. It seems that those cultures that live the longest have a wonderful sense of community. Several generations live in the vicinity of each other. The elderly, young, and middle-aged all interact on a regular basis. There seems to be caring and consideration for everyone in the community. The older people are revered for their wisdom. There is a sense of cooperation and teamwork. There is a feeling that for one to succeed, all must succeed. In these societies there are strong religious beliefs. There is a belief that there is something or someone bigger than themselves, to whom people must account in the final analysis. This belief helps people to make good decisions for themselves and others. These people work hard together and play hard together.

Group goals and individual goals give people something to look forward to. It is hard to feel depressed about your own life if your focus is outside yourself. Being helpful, loving, and supportive of others is a wonderful cure for depression.

I understand that we live in the twenty-first century, and a lot of us don't have close families or communities. Many of us have lost our mothers or fathers. There is a feeling of disconnectedness. If we have living relatives, they may live far away or may be so wrapped up in their own lives that it seems impossible to connect. Fortunately, we have the power as human beings to create our own families. You know the folks in your life who make you feel celebrated instead of tolerated. Make those persons part of your new family. Surround yourself with people you love, admire, and respect. Make their concerns and goals your concerns and goals. Develop personal integrity by being as honest as you can without hurting others.

Many people have some religious beliefs. Even if people do not believe in a god, they know right from wrong. If a people get involved in community service or volunteer work, it enhances their lives. There is something about helping folks who are in need that does wonders for your sense of purpose.

It is important to maintain an attitude of gratitude. This means focusing on those things in your life that are positive. Celebrate the things that you have, instead of bemoaning those things you don't have. When you have an attitude of gratitude, it is almost impossible to feel fear, resentment, sorrow, or a sense of hopelessness.

Making short- and long-term attainable goals is a good way to make sure you have something to look forward to and something to work toward. Find out what your gifts or strengths are, and try to perfect them.

Looking at the wonders of nature is a great way to feel a sense of awe and appreciation of the world around you. Geese in flight, a beautiful horse running, the Grand Canyon, among other things, have to make you feel a sense of wonder about the world you live in, and at the same time, seeing them can be very relaxing.

Using yoga or breathing techniques to learn how to relax can be quite helpful. Most people are shallow breathers. Try taking a big breath to the count of ten, hold it for a count of eight, and then release it for a count of six, exhaling through the mouth. Repeat at least ten times. If you try this before going to bed or whenever you feel stressed, you'll find it very relaxing.

It has been proven that having a pet is very therapeutic. Animals tend to soothe a person. Having a pet to care for and love can be very beneficial.

Chapter 7: Special Areas of Concern to Fliers

Varicose Veins[1]

When preparing to write this book, I asked my flying partners what their issues were. A great many of them complained of varicose veins. I was surprised to learn that more men than women had varicose vein concerns.

Just what are varicose veins? They are large, twisted veins, usually in the legs and feet, that are not transporting blood effectively. They look like bulging, bluish cords beneath the surface of the skin. If not treated, varicose veins can cause not only discomfort and cosmetic concerns, but also complications such as phlebitis, skin ulcers, and blood clots.

Signs of Varicose Veins

Some signs of varicose veins are the following: swelling in the ankles and feet, especially after standing; prominent dark blue blood vessels in the legs and feet; and aching, tender, heavy, or sore legs. There may be breaks in the skin and superficial blood clots. There can be bleeding after a minor injury.

Causes of Varicose Veins

Varicose veins happen when the veins stretch and their valves, which usually prevent the backflow of blood, fail. Primary varicose veins result from weakness in the walls of the veins. Primary varicose veins result from congenitally defective valves or without a known cause. Secondary varicose occur because of some other condition, such as when a pregnant woman develops varicose veins. Secondary varicose veins are most often lying deep beneath, among the muscles, which carry about 90 percent of the returning blood to the heart. Some problems include blood clots and the resulting diversion of blood flow into the other superficial vessels.

Who Is Most at Risk for Varicose Veins

Family history is a 50 percent cause. People who have a parent with varicose veins, have a fifty percent risk of getting varicose veins also. Females are more at risk. Hormonal changes related to pregnancy, to the time period just before menstruation, and to menopause are another risk factor. Standing for long periods of time will put you at risk. Obesity and tumors can contribute to your risk for varicose veins. Abnormal blood flow between arteries and veins is another contributor.

Prevention and Treatment of Varicose Veins

Regular exercise improves vein function and promotes weight loss. Avoid prolonged sitting, standing, or walking; get regular exercise; elevate legs on a periodic basis; and wear compression stockings. Eating foods rich in dietary fiber in the form of complex carbohydrates and bioflavonoides (found in dark leafy green vegetables, garlic, onions, citrus fruits, and some other fruits) may prove helpful for the prevention of varicose veins, recovery from them, and prevention of recurrences.

Herbs That May Aid Recovery from Varicose Veins

Note: Check with your medical doctor before using these or any herbs, as they are not appropriate for all people.

- Horse chestnut (*Aesculus hippocastanum*), between 300 mg tablets, 3 times daily.

  For centuries, horse chestnut seeds, leaves, bark, and flowers have been used for a variety of conditions and diseases. Horse chestnut seed extract has been used to treat chronic venous insufficiency (a condition in which the veins do not efficiently return blood from the legs to the heart). This condition is associated with varicose veins, pain, ankle swelling, feelings of heaviness, itching, and nighttime leg cramping. The seed extract has also been used for hemorrhoids.

  See more information at: http://nccam.nih.gov/health/horsechestnut/

- Butcher's broom *(Ruscus aculeatus),* 100 mg tablets, 3 times a day.

  Butcher's broom has been known to enhance blood flow to the brain, legs, and hands. It has been used to relieve constipation and water retention and improve circulation. Since Butcher's broom tightens blood vessels and capillaries, it is used to treat a common condition known as varicose veins (Bouskela , Cyrino, and Marcelon). Butcher's broom seems to have a favorable effect on the legs. Veins constrict after consumption of the herb and swelling subsides. By acting directly on the blood vessels, butcher's broom increases blood flow and thus an increase in circulation is precipitated. Butcher's broom has been used as a diuretic in folk medicine and was believed to be a mild osmotic diuretic: a substance which draws water out of cells. Some people who consume butcher's broom capsules do in fact notice a urinary output increase.

  See more details at: http://www.vitawise.com/butcbroo.htm

- Gotu kola *(Centella asiatica),* 500 mg tablets, 2 to 4 times daily

  Gotu kola is also used topically as an ointment to treat a variety of skin conditions. UMM says that it contains chemicals called triterpenoids which have antioxidant properties that help to heal wounds and minor burns and to prevent scarring after an injury or surgery. Due to the triterpenoids it may also help to strengthen the skin, increase blood flow to it, and consequently to treat skin disorders such as acne and psoriasis. In addition, gotu kola may be beneficial for the prevention and reduction of stretch marks. Balch warns however in that certain individual's gotu kola may cause dermatitis when applied topically. According to the American Cancer Society, some preliminary clinical trials have found that gotu kola may improve poor blood flow to the legs and help to reduce swelling. Individuals with a condition called chronic venous insufficiency, characterized by swelling of the legs and feet due to varicose veins and poor circulation, were given an extract of gotu kola. The gotu kola extract seemed to reduce the leakage of blood vessels that contribute to swelling, and the herb was deemed more helpful than the placebo. The American Cancer Society warns however that more research needs to be done, and herbs do not always produce the same benefits as extracts made from them Read more: http://www.livestrong.com/article/388873-benefits-uses-for-gotu-kola/

Another remedy to be used topically is: Combine the following equal parts: yarrow, hawthorn, ginkgo, ginger, and horse chestnut into a tincsure. Take thirty to sixty drops of the tincture two to three times daily, or drink three to four cups of the tea daily. Cold compresses of witch hazel and yarrow tea may provide relief.

Hearing Loss

Many of my flying partners have experienced hearing loss and ear pain or discomfort from flying. I was once stranded in Boston with a ruptured eardrum. It was a painful and time-consuming experience. I could not fly home. I had to take a five-day trip on Amtrak to get home.

First off, please don't fly with a sinus infection or head cold; you're asking for trouble. If you must fly, take Sudafed or another decongestant beforehand. I don't recommend taking Sudafed for long periods, as it may cause your heart to race.

There have been many studies by the military that evaluated the risk of hearing loss among its fliers. Descriptive data includes time-weighted average noise exposure and elevation of groups of flight personnel. They found that the more workdays fliers had, the greater their hearing loss was.

When you are feeling discomfort, you need to know what is happening. The external pressure on your body is increasing because the cabin is pressurized, but the pressure on your inner ear is sealed from the outside and does not change. This causes the eardrum to bulge inward and results in a loss of hearing. This also causes pain and discomfort. If you pinch your nose and blow lightly you can sometimes minimize the pain. Another remedy is to chew gum. If you cover the ear with a wet, warm cloth that has been drained of water, you can sometimes send steam into the ear to help equalize the pressure in the eustachian tube.

EARS AND MOTION SICKNESS

You may feel motion sickness in your belly, but it starts in your inner ear. The balance hubs in the ear can be thrown off by turbulence or whenever what you see (a stable cabin) doesn't match what you feel (in flight motion). Your best prevention, book a seat over the wings, the most stable part of the plane. To add insult to injury, those tunes you're blasting to block the engine noise are weakening your ears nerve cells. Your hearing won't take a long term hit after a plane ride or two, but if you're a frequent flyer, you could be setting yourself up for permanent damage.

Source; Phyllis Kozarsky MD,
Travelers Branch, US Centers for
Disease Control and Prevention

Carpal Tunnel Syndrome

According to Dr. Robert (Bob) Marshall of Premier Research Labs, carpal tunnel syndrome is caused by compression of the median nerve that travels through the carpal tunnel, a narrow passageway located on the palm side of your wrist. It affects the main nerve to the hand and results in motor and sensory disturbance. This condition causes pain, weakness, and sometimes paralysis in the median nerve. One may have tingling, numbness, and pain sensations throughout the arm; the feelings can travel to the shoulder and neck. This syndrome may be more prevalent at night due to sleeping positions. Stretching exercises or night splints to stabilize and support joints may be helpful.

Carpal tunnel syndrome is linked to infection in the joints, low pH, toxic liver, deficient minerals, deficient vitamin B, and weak adrenals.

It can be caused by pressure on the median nerve, obesity, diabetes, hypothyroidism, arthritis, and trauma. Benign tumors can also be a cause.

Internal pressure as well as pressure on the medial nerve from sources outside your hand can be the cause of carpal tunnel syndrome. Repetitive motions can cause carpal tunnel syndrome. Awkward postures and vibrations on a moving aircraft can cause stress to the muscles and can contribute to carpal tunnel syndrome. Since a flight attendant has to push and pull four-hundred-pound liquor carts, it is easy to understand why so many of my coworkers suffer from carpal tunnel syndrome. The repetitive motion of the hand can result in permanent damage.

Some people have suggested that reducing the amount of red meat, dairy, refined foods, and soft drinks you take in and eating more vegetables will help relieve the condition. A person suffering from carpal tunnel syndrome should exercise the upper arms daily.

Health Tips for Fliers

* If you are going to travel, always carry any medications you may need with you. Make sure you are prepared for any possible delays. If you have allergies, wear a medical alert bracelet and carry the name and phone number of your doctor.

* Be very careful to keep hydrated and avoid caffeinated drinks.

* Exercise as much as possible while away.

* Try not to fly if you have a sinus or ear infection. The pressurization of the cabin during flight can aggravate these conditions.

* If for any reason you need to take oxygen, know that the airlines provide this service. For those of you who scuba dive, plan to travel twelve to twenty-four hours after your dive.

* There are many destinations you may fly to that require vaccinations. Some vaccinations take up to six weeks to be effective. Give yourself plenty of time before your flight to receive your vaccinations.

* Always be sure to have copies of any dental and physical exams with you before you fly. You should make sure you have enough cash and credit cards to pay for any medical attention you may need. A great many countries will not honor insurance cards.

* It is a good idea not to eat at street markets or from street vendors, or you could risk parasites. Be careful what you eat. All meals should be well cooked. Please make sure the bottles you drink from are sealed. Make certain you brush your teeth with bottled water. Be certain that you peel any fruits you eat.

* If you are going to an exotic location, have insect repellent and try to sleep in a netted area. Avoid swimming in streams, ponds, or lakes. You don't know what kind of bugs are there.

* If you plan on renting a car or motorbike, try not to drive at night. If possible, get a map and learn the local rules of the road.

* Hand sanitizers, nail clippers, and a thermometer are good to have along with you. You could also use tweezers, scissors, and bandages.

* If you take prescription medications, carry them in their original containers. Make sure you have painkillers, decongestants, and antihistamines for allergies. Sunscreen and antibacterial salves can also prove handy. If you are prone to motion sickness, bring Dramamine.

* There is nothing more frustrating than, after a long day of travel, arriving at your hotel starving, only to find out that room service is closed and there is no place to eat. My favorite tip is to carry plenty of healthy snacks. I like to keep power bars handy. Fresh fruits and vegetables are always a good snack, as are fresh raw nuts, raisins, and boiled eggs. Organic peanut butter and crackers are quite tasty. Packages of instant oatmeal pack well, as do cheese and crackers.

LAVATORY HINTS

Do you have to use the lavatory in flight? So would someone suffering from norovirus, a powerful and super contagious cause of diarrhea and vomiting. It can live on bathroom faucets and door handles and even tray tables. Swabbing these areas with an alcohol based wipe can help, so keep using hand sanitizer after touching anything communal.

How to Degerm a Hotel Room.

It's a good idea to pack a travel –size Lysol disinfectant spray. Upon entering your hotel room, wash your hands, you've probably turned a doorknob, pushed an elevator button, and handled money. Up to 80% of infections are transmitted by hands, and a ton of other people, so it's important to eliminate any potential pathogens on your hands before you contaminate everything else in the room. Don't eat, drink or touch your face until you've washed up.

What next? inspect the room, starting with the bathroom, which is the biggest source of germs. With a tissue, lift the toilet seat and spray both sides of the seat with Lysol, even if it looks spotless. Wash glasses or mugs with hand soap and hot water if they're not sealed in a wrapper, and leave them open side up to dry. The same goes for ice buckets without plastic liners. Next, use wipes on frequently touched hot spots; faucets, the toilet lever, doorknobs, light switches, the phone, clock radio and especially the TV remote.

Don't sit or place any belonging on the bed until you're sure it's parasite-free. Peel back the fitted sheet and examine the mattress for bedbugs or signs of them. Alert management right away if you spot dried blood stains, tiny white eggs, or bedbug skin or cells, which are often transparent or pale yellow. If there is a bedspread, put it away in a corner. It's unlikely to have been washed or changed recently. Leave a note for housekeeping to not make the bed with the bedspread during your stay. A duvet tends to be safer, but keep the top sheet between you and the cover and fold the sheet over the edge so your chin is protected.

Other areas you should avoid; Keep your hands off the drapes. They trap a lot of dust and allergens and gems build up over time. Also limit contact with the carpets and furniture so you don't pick up any potential fungus. That means you should wear socks or slippers and be fully clothed when sitting on the furniture.

It is a nice idea to place Bounce fabric sheets on the mattress to ward off bed bugs and in/around your luggage to keep away bugs.

Before bathing squirt shampoo in the tub and run hot water for a minute to decrease the number of germs where you'll be standing. As long as you don't have abrasions on your feet, it's not likely that you'll contract something. If you have a cut on the foot, though, bandage it and wear flip flops. As for taking a bath, you may want to skip that entirely during your stay due to biofilm, a nearly undetectable layer of bacteria that sticks to tubs and other surfaces. It comes off only with vigorous scrubbing with a hard-bristle brush and soap.

What is the worse illness you can contact from hotel-room germs? You could catch anything from a norovirus to a cold to a staph skin infection. Most of the time you'll walk away completely fine. It all depends on what type of germs the previous guests left behind and how well the room was cleaned.

How can you make sure the room you're booking is clean? People think a higher-end hotel guarantees cleanliness, but that's not always the case. There can be housekeeping staffers who cut corners in any hotel. The best thing you can do is read lodging reviews online. Specific feedback and photos from former guests are more helpful than star ratings; if other customers experience dirty sheets or a grimy tub, you may encounter the same during your stay.

Reference: Microbiologist Phillip M. Tierno, PHD a professor of microbiology at NEW YORK UNIVERSITY OF MEDICINE< in NEW YORK CITY

Conclusion

This world of ours can be a beautiful place, but there are many elements about it that can harm us if we are not diligent. Toxins are everywhere: gas fumes, electromagnetic fields, over processed foods, pesticides, and preservatives, to name a few. It's said that the body you have at twenty years of age is the body God gave you and the body you have at fifty years of age is the one you gave yourself. This body we have is a gift that must be nurtured. It is a fabulous machine, unlike any other.

Because there are many hazards out there, we must be careful what we place in and on our bodies. We must be good stewards of the gifts we have been given. As I said before, taking care of our health is the only investment we can make that pays dividends. We don't know how long we will live, but we all can have a say in the quality of that life.

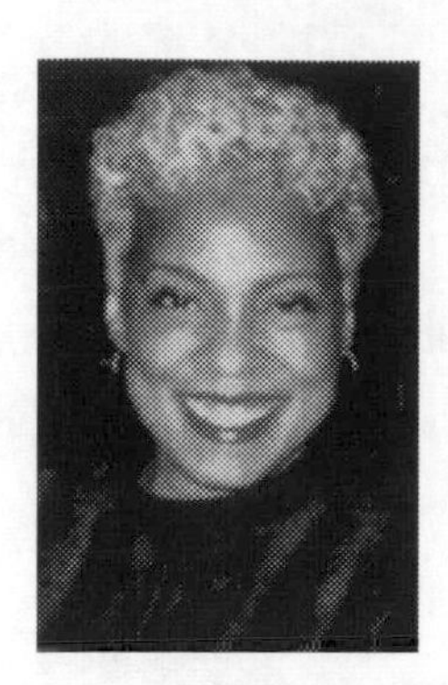

About the Author

Stephanie Coleman is a native of Chicago, Illinois. She is a certified nutrition consultant, a certified reflexologist, and a certified natural health professional. Stephanie has been a flight attendant for over thirty-eight years. Her love of travel and airplanes led her to become a private pilot. She has been licensed since 1979. Stephanie received a bachelor's degree in 1996 and is an accomplished artist.

Stephanie is the mother of an Air Force major, also a pilot. Stephanie's father was a Tuskegee airman, and her husband was a Navy pilot. Over the years, she has come in contact with a lot of airline and military people.

Stephanie is a breast cancer survivor.

With the experience of having cancer and seeing how victims of cancer are treated, she has developed a strong interest in most health issues, as well as a continuing thirst for health knowledge. Stephanie realizes how little the average American knows about the workings and needs of their own bodies. This book is an attempt to inform the general public, as well as airline employees, of what they can do to be proactive about their own health and to prevent disease when they fly.

REFERENCES

Introduction

1. http://www.justmeans.com/press-releases/Kaiser-Permanente-Seniors-and-Boomers-Discover-Key-to-Stayin g-Young-and-Healthy/7535.html accessed on 11/20/2010. (1)

2. www.healthcareproblems.org (2, 5 and 6)

3. www.aoa.gov/ Administration on Aging (3)

4. www.kff.org - *You +1'd this publicly.* Undo

5. *The* Kaiser Family Foundation (4, 7, 8, 14 and 15)

6. www.who.int/research/en/ - World Health Organization (9 and 10)

7. http://2010.census.gov/2010census/ - People and households (10 and 13)

8. www.ebri.org/.../facts/?...fastfacts - EBRI – Employee Benefit Research Institute (16 and 17)

Chapter 1:

1. Day, Phillip, *Health Wars* - Credence Publications, Kent, UK (2001), pg. 183 - 186. (1 – 13)

2. Marshall, Robert – QRA (Quantum Reflex Analysis) – Seminar conducted on June, 29, 2008 (14 – 23)

3. W. Friedberg, K. Copeland, F. E. Duke, K. O'Brien III and E. B. Darden, Jr. - Radiation Exposure During Air Travel: Guidance Provided by the Federal Aviation Administration for Air Carrier Crews accessed on June 18, 2010. (24-30) http://www.faa.gov/data_research/research/med_humanfacs/aeromedical/radiobiology/reports/

4. John P. Cunha, "Jet Lag," MedicineNet.com, accessed April 27, 2011, (31 – 43) http://www.medicinenet.com/jet_lag/article.htm#1whatis – jet lag.

Chapter 2

1. Phillip Day, *Health Wars,* PO Box 3 Tonbridge KENT tn12 9zy UK Credence Publications, (2001), pg 204–212 (1 – 10)

2. Marshall, Robert – QRA (Quantum Reflex Analysis) – Seminar conducted on June 29, 2008 (11 – 13, 50 – 53 and 56 – 57)

3. Mercola, Joseph. Soft drinks and diseases, accessed on December 2, 2010 from an article reproduced at http://

www.mindconnection.com/library/health/softdrinks.htm 33. (14 - 32)

4. Smoking - http://quitsmoking.about.com/od/tobaccostatistics/a/CigaretteSmoke.htm (33 – 49)

5. Chi and Meridian concepts – accessed on September 12, 2010 at http://www.aworldofchinesemedicine.com/ (54 – 55)

6. Taylor, Nadine, *Green Tea: The Natural Secret for a Healthier Life* (New York: Kensington Publishing Corporation, 1998). (56 – 67)

7. Daniels, Stephen. Green Tea's Alzheimer protection gets more support. (2008) accessed on December 1, 2010 at claims that the beverage may help ward off Alzheimer's. (68 – 71) http://www.nutraingredients.com/Research/Green-tea-s-Alzheimer-protection-gets-more-support

8. Life Extension Article "Cancer radiation therapy" accessed on September 5 2010 at http://www.lef.org/protocols/cancer/radiation_therapy_01.htm (72)

9. Warner, Jennifer. Green Tea Ingredient may promote healthy weight loss, accessed on June 05, 2010 at http://www.webmd.com/diet/news/20050126/green-tea-fights-fat (73)

Chapter 3:

1. "Your Bodies Many Cries For Water" by F.Batmanghelidj, MD. Publisher Global Health Solutions INC April 2008 USA (1). pg 152-153 (2-4). pg 106-108 (5). Pg36-37

2. www.European Hydration Institute.org (6-9) "Home Grown Kids" by Raymond and Dorthy Moore pg 113

3. www.Symptoms of Dehydration.com (10-14) accessed on July 14, 2010.

Chapter 4:

1. Elaine Newkirk, "Basic Nutrition" (lecture notes, Nutrition: Nov 2008) Trinity School of Natural Health, 10 South Buffalo Street Warsaw, Indiana 46580. (1-14)

2. Mia Scheid, CNC, Mias@fitnessarts.net (15 -17)

Chapter 5:

1. Lecture notes, Nutrtion Consultant Certification, Global College of Natural Medicine, 250 Natural Bridges Dr. Santa Cruz, CA.GCNM.Com(1-5)

Chapter 6:

1. Phillip Day, Health Wars Credence Publications , PO Box 3 Tonbridge, Kent TN12 9ZY Uk 2007(1)

Chapter 7:

1. Bob Marshall (lecture notes), Premier Research Labs Quantum Nutrition Labs. Level 1 .July 15 2007 Chicago, Ill

2. Mia Scheid, CNC, Mias@fitnessarts.net

3. Aerospace Medical Association, **"Tips for Healthy Comfortable Air Travel" Acessed November 20, 2010,** http://www.asma.org/pdf/publications/tips_for_travelers.pdf - Association

Printed in the United States
By Bookmasters